Master the Art of Romantic Sex

An A-Z Guide to a Wonderful Sexual Experience

plus Tips for Couples to Make Sex More

Romantic and Intimate

Cheryl Bach

Master the Art of Romantic Sex

Cheryl Bach

Table of Contents

Cheryl Bach

I.

Introduction

Importance of Romantic and Intimate Sex

Sex is a natural and beautiful aspect of our lives that can bring us pleasure, intimacy, and connection with our partners. However, many couples struggle to maintain a satisfying and fulfilling sex life over time. Often, couples find themselves falling into routines or becoming disconnected, which can lead to feelings of dissatisfaction, boredom, and even resentment in some cases.

This is where the importance of romantic and intimate sex comes in. Romantic sex isn't just about roses, candles, and soft music, but it is rather an approach to sex that emphasizes closeness, connection, and tenderness between partners. It's about creating a unique and special bond between you and your partner that elevates your relationship to another level.

The Benefits of Incorporating Romance into Your Sex Life

The benefits of incorporating romance into your sex life are numerous. Studies show that couples who incorporate romance into their sex lives report higher levels of relationship satisfaction and intimacy. Additionally, it can help strengthen the emotional connection between partners and increase feelings of love and affection. Romantic sex can also help to reduce negative feelings and conflicts that arise in relationships, which can lead to a more fulfilling sex life.

Cheryl Bach

Overview of the Book

This book, "Master the Art of Romantic Sex: An A-Z Guide to a Wonderful Sexual Experience plus Tips for Couples to Make Sex More Romantic and Intimate," is designed to help couples achieve a more satisfying and fulfilling sex life by incorporating romantic and intimate elements into their sexual experiences.

Throughout this book, we will explore a variety of techniques, tips, and strategies to help you and your partner improve your sex life. The book covers everything from creating the perfect ambiance to exploring each other's desires, from extended and varied foreplay to using jewelry, kinks, tantra, and other methods to enhance the intimacy and pleasure of sexual experiences

Together, we will explore how to maintain intimacy, discuss fantasies and desires, communicate openly with each other, and try new things to keep your sexual relationship fresh and exciting. We will also focus on the importance of emotional connection and ways to initiate and explore new experiences together.

By implementing these tools and techniques, you can cultivate a more loving and satisfying connection with your partner, which will enhance your overall relationship and boost your sexual experiences.

Throughout the rest of the book, we'll cover topics such as the power of sensual massage, the role of oral sex, incorporating playfulness in the bedroom, the benefits of tantric practices, and tips for keeping things fresh and exciting between the sheets regardless of how long you have been partners.

So whether you've been in a relationship for several years or are just starting out, this book will give you the tools you need to elevate your sexual experiences to a new level of intimacy and fulfillment.

We invite you to read this book with an open mind and to be willing to experiment, explore, and learn with your partner. With the right mindset and willingness, this journey can lead to a more fulfilling and pleasurable sex life for both partners.

Remember that it takes effort, practice, and open communication to maintain a healthy and satisfying sexual connection. But with the insights and techniques in this book, you'll be well on your way to mastering the art of romantic sex and experiencing a more fulfilling, intimate, and loving relationship with your partner.

Let's dive in and explore what it means to truly master the art of romantic sex.

Cheryl Bach

II.

A - Z Guide to Romantic Sex

In this chapter, we'll dive into an A-Z guide that covers everything you need to know about mastering the art of romantic and intimate sex. By exploring each concept, you can learn how to create a deeper sense of connection and intimacy in your sexual relationship with your partner.

A. Ambiance - How to Create the Perfect Atmosphere

Creating the right atmosphere can be crucial to setting the mood for romantic sex. Start by dimming the lights and using candles or fairy lights to create a soft and sensual ambiance. You can also use background music to set the tone. Make sure to keep the room free of distractions such as electronics, and turn off your phone. Additionally, consider getting a high-quality, comfortable bed that provides a balanced level of support.

B. Body Language - Using Non-Verbal Cues to Communicate

Body language is a critical part of communication, even during sex. Practice using non-verbal cues such as eye contact, touch, and body positioning to communicate your desires and feelings. Pay attention to your partner's body language and respond accordingly.

C. Communication - Open and Honest Communication to Increase Intimacy

Communication is key to building a deeper connection and increasing intimacy in your relationship. Be open and honest with your partner about your feelings, desires, and boundaries. Remember, communication is not just verbal but can also be through body language and touch.

D. Desire - Exploring Each Other's Desires

Understanding and exploring each other's desires can help create a more fulfilling sexual experience for both partners. Take the time to ask your partner about their fantasies and desires and share your own. Experiment and try new things together, with both partners feeling safe and comfortable in exploring their desires.

E. Foreplay - Tips for Extended and Varied Foreplay

Foreplay can be a critically important part of creating an intimate and satisfying sexual experience. Explore different forms of foreplay such as kissing, touching, and oral sex. Take the time to slowly build arousal and make sure both partners are fully prepared for intercourse.

F. Grooming - Personal Grooming and Hygiene

Personal grooming and hygiene are key to feeling confident and comfortable during sex. Make sure to maintain good hygiene, including regular showering and shaving. Consider grooming your pubic hair to your and you partner's liking.

G. Healthy Relationship - Building a Healthy Romantic Relationship

A healthy relationship creates a foundation of trust, respect, and communication that makes romantic sex more fulfilling. Take the time to work on your relationship outside of the bedroom by building meaningful experiences together and fostering open and honest communication.

H. Intimacy - How to Increase and Maintain Intimacy

Intimacy is more than just physical touch - it's about feeling emotionally connected with your partner. Take the time to create a sense of emotional intimacy by talking about your feelings, dreams, and desires. Additionally, use physical touch outside of sexual contexts, such as cuddling or holding hands, to build connection.

I. Jewelry - Ways to Incorporate Jewelry into Sex Play

Jewelry can be used to add an additional level of sensuality to your sexual experience. Consider wearing jewelry during sex play, or even using it to stimulate certain areas of the body during foreplay.

J. Kink - Exploring Kinks in a Romantic Way

Exploring kinks can be a great way to add novelty and excitement to your sex life. However, it's important to make sure both partners feel safe and comfortable during any kink-related activities. Communicate with your partner about their interests and boundaries, and consider starting small with something like light bondage or role-playing before exploring more intense kinks.

K. Lingerie - Wearing Lingerie to Enhance the Sexual Experience

Lingerie can help you feel confident and sensual during sex. Consider wearing lingerie that makes you feel sexy and comfortable to help set the mood and add an additional level of intimacy to your sexual experience.

L. Masturbation - Benefits of Masturbation for a Healthy Sex Life

Masturbation can be a healthy way to explore your own body and desires, and can even improve your sex life with a partner by helping you communicate your needs and desires better. Don't be afraid to share your masturbation habits with your partner and incorporate it into your sexual routine if it feels comfortable and pleasurable for both of you.

Cheryl Bach

C. The Importance of Emotional Connection

Emotional connection is crucial for building intimacy in a relationship both inside and outside of the bedroom. Communicate openly and honestly with your partner about your thoughts, feelings, and desires, and take time to actively listen and understand their perspective. Building an emotional connection outside of the bedroom will lead to greater intimacy inside the bedroom.

D. Encouraging Open and Honest Communication

To create a deeper emotional connection and make sex more romantic and intimate, it's important for couples to communicate openly and honestly. Be open and transparent about your desires, feelings, and boundaries. Encourage your partner to do the same. Make sure to listen attentively and respond respectfully to ensure that both partners feel comfortable and heard. This type of communication can help build trust and strengthen the emotional bonds between partners.

Master the Art of Romantic Sex

E. Ways to Initiate and Explore New Experiences Together

Trying new things together can help improve intimacy in a relationship. Experiment with different techniques, positions, toys, or media, but be sure to respect each other's boundaries and comfort levels. Find ways to initiate new experiences together by suggesting fantasies, sharing erotica, or taking a sex education class. By exploring new things together, couples can create excitement and anticipation around their sexual experiences which leads to greater intimacy.

F. Discussing Fantasies and Desires with One Another

Sharing fantasies and desires with your partner can help create a deeper emotional connection and make sex more romantic and intimate. Talk openly about your desires and ask your partner about theirs. Be sure to express what you're comfortable with and set boundaries, so that both partners feel safe and heard. When discussing fantasies and desires, be patient and respectful with your partner's responses. This type of communication can lead to shared experiences that bring couples closer together.

G. The Benefits of Trying New Things Together

Trying new experiences together can be beneficial for relationships in many ways. It can lead to increased intimacy and trust, as well as help couples better understand their own sexual preferences. Additionally, exploring new things together can help reignite passion in a long-term relationship and prevent boredom or monotony in the bedroom.

Cheryl Bach

IV.

How to Maintain a Strong and Satisfying Sex Life Long-Term

Maintaining a strong and satisfying sex life long-term can be a challenge for many couples. The initial spark of passion can slowly fade away over time, leaving couples feeling unfulfilled and unsatisfied. However, there are ways to keep the heat alive in your relationship and maintain a healthy, satisfying sex life over the years.

A. The Importance of Keeping Things Fresh and Exciting

Maintaining a strong and satisfying sex life long-term requires a willingness to keep things fresh and exciting. It can be easy to fall into a routine where the same sexual techniques are used all the time, leading to decreased arousal and a lack of excitement in the bedroom. This is why it's important to mix things up and try new things.

One way to keep things fresh and exciting is to experiment with new sexual positions. If you always have sex in the same position, try adding in a different position to spice things up. Role-playing is another fun way to bring excitement into the bedroom. Costumes and acting out scenarios can be a great way to bring some newness into the relationship.

B. Using Feedback to Improve Your Sex Life

Feedback is essential to keeping a strong and satisfying sex life. It's important to communicate with your partner and ask for feedback on what he or she likes and dislikes. This can be done through verbal communication or through physical cues such as moans and movements.

Cheryl Bach

E. Incorporating Daily Acts of Affection

Daily acts of affection can enhance intimacy and strengthen the emotional connection between partners. Small acts of affection such as holding hands, hugging, kissing, and cuddling can help build intimacy and create a sense of closeness outside of the bedroom.

It's important to incorporate daily acts of affection into your routine even if you're busy. Even something as simple as leaving a sweet note in your partner's lunch or sending a quick message during the day can make a big difference in maintaining a strong and satisfying sex life long-term.

F. Keeping the Romance and Intimacy Alive Over Time

Keeping the romance and intimacy alive over time requires creativity and effort. It's important to continue to date each other and plan romantic outings together such as dinners, weekend getaways, or couples massages.

Master the Art of Romantic Sex

In addition to this, it's important to continue to prioritize physical touch and intimacy outside of sex. This helps to build anticipation and excitement that can carry over into the bedroom.

Lastly, don't forget to surprise your partner with small gestures of affection. This could be anything from a surprise gift to a loving gesture or act of service that shows your partner how much you care.

By keeping the romance and intimacy alive over time, you can ensure that your sex life stays strong and satisfying for years to come.

In conclusion, maintaining a strong and satisfying sex life long-term requires effort, commitment, and communication between partners. By keeping things fresh and exciting, using feedback to improve your sex life, communicating sexual needs and desires effectively, understanding the importance of consistency and commitment, incorporating daily acts of affection and keeping the romance and intimacy alive over time, you can keep your sex life healthy and satisfying for both you and your partner.

Cheryl Bach

𝒱.

Conclusion

A. Summary of the Key Takeaways of Mastering the Art of Romantic Sex

Throughout this book, we've covered a variety of topics related to mastering the art of romantic sex. From communication and experimentation to techniques for building intimacy and making sex more romantic, the key takeaway is that a strong and satisfying sex life requires effort, openness, and a willingness to try new things.

Some of the key takeaways from this book include the importance of communication and feedback in creating a healthy sexual relationship, the role of intimacy and romance in enhancing pleasure and satisfaction, and the need for exploration and experimentation when it comes to sexual techniques and positions.

In summary, mastering the art of romantic sex involves creating a safe and open environment where both partners feel comfortable sharing their desires and needs, and both are committed to exploring and growing in their sexual relationship.

B. Final Thoughts and Encouragement for Couples to Continue Exploring and Growing in Their Sex Lives

As couples continue to explore and grow in their sexual relationship, it's important to remember that sex should be enjoyable and satisfying for both partners. Don't be afraid to try new things or experiment with different techniques and positions.

It's also important to prioritize intimacy and romance outside of the bedroom. By incorporating acts of affection into your daily routine, planning romantic outings, and keeping the relationship fresh and exciting, you can maintain a healthy and satisfying sex life over time.

Remember that communication and feedback are key in keeping the spark alive and creating a strong sexual connection with your partner. Don't be afraid to share your desires and needs, and encourage your partner to do the same.

C. Additional Resources for Further Exploration and Learning

If you're interested in learning more about mastering the art of romantic sex, there are a variety of resources available to you.

Here are a few recommended options:

Sex Therapy: If you're experiencing sexual problems or difficulties in your relationship, consider working with a sex therapist who can help you identify and address the underlying issues.

Books and Literature: There are many books available that offer advice and guidance on romantic sex, including "Come As You Are" by Emily Nagoski, "The Mult-Orgasmic Couple" by Mantak Chia and Maneewan Chia, and "The 5 Love Languages" by Gary Chapman.

Workshops and Classes: Many communities have sex-positive workshops and classes that focus on communication, intimacy, and sexual techniques. These can be a great way to learn new skills and connect with like-minded individuals.

Online Resources: There are many online communities and resources focused on sexual education and exploration. These include websites, blogs, forums, and social media groups where you can connect with others who share your interests and learn new techniques and tips.

Couples Retreats: Consider attending a couples retreat, where you and your partner can work with experts in the field of romantic sex to deepen your connection and explore new ways of enhancing pleasure and satisfaction.

By exploring these resources and continuing to grow and learn together, you and your partner can master the art of romantic sex and enjoy a fulfilling and satisfying sex life for years to come.

In conclusion, mastering the art of romantic sex is about creating a healthy and open environment where both partners feel comfortable sharing their desires and needs. By prioritizing intimacy, communication, and experimentation, you can enhance pleasure and satisfaction in your sexual relationship. Remember that there are many resources available to you, and don't be afraid to seek out the support and guidance of experts in the field, such as sex therapists and couples retreats. Through ongoing exploration and learning, you can create a strong and satisfying sexual connection that enhances your overall relationship with your partner.

By prioritizing intimacy, communication, and new experiences, you can create a sex life that is fulfilling and satisfying for both partners. Remember to keep an open and honest approach to communication, have a curious mindset when it comes to trying new things, and prioritize intimacy and romance outside of the bedroom to create a healthy and thriving sexual relationship.

Thank you for reading "Master the Art of Romantic Sex: An A-Z Guide to a Wonderful Sexual Experience plus Tips for Couples to Make Sex More Romantic and Intimate." We wish you the best of luck in your journey towards mastering the art of romantic sex and encourage you to continue exploring and growing in your sexual relationship. Remember that every couple's journey is unique, and what works for one may not work for another. Embrace your individuality as a couple and be willing to try new things to find what works best for you.

Finally, never forget the importance of consent and respect in any sexual situation. Always prioritize the comfort and safety of both partners and practice safe sex to protect against sexually transmitted infections and unwanted pregnancies.

With these principles in mind and a commitment to ongoing growth and exploration, you can create a truly wonderful and fulfilling sexual experience with your partner.

www.ingramcontent.com/pod-product-compliance
Lightning Source LLC
Chambersburg PA
CBHW051712250726
48653CB00007B/2985